LET'S CELEBRATE YOUR STORY

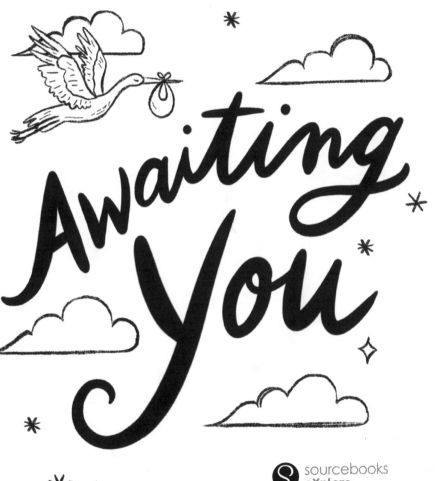

Awaiting You

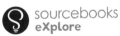

sourcebooks eXplore

A PREGNANCY JOURNAL

To the boy in my belly while I wrote.
The bigger you grew, Linden, the deeper I fell in love.

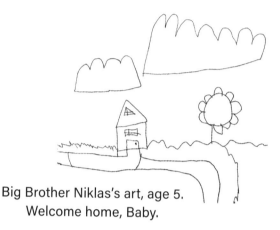

Big Brother Niklas's art, age 5.
Welcome home, Baby.

Published by Sourcebooks eXplore, an imprint of Sourcebooks Kids
P.O. Box 4410, Naperville, Illinois 60567-4410
(630) 961-3900
sourcebooks.com

Originally published in 2017 in the United States of America by Katie Clemons LLC.

Printed and bound in the United States of America.

VP 10 9 8 7 6 5 4 3 2 1

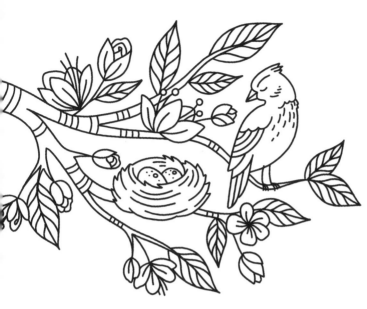

CRAFT your BIRDSONG

ON A COOL SUMMER EVENING when bluebirds twittered in the trees and my pregnant belly was just beginning to swell over my shorts, I watched my husband, Martin, punching numbers into a scientific calculator.

Wow, I still remember wanting to interrupt. *We're having a baby! I can't wait to kiss his soft cheeks.*

I knew Martin would stop doing homework, rub my belly, and grin in agreement, just as he'd done the half-million other times I'd interjected with baby thoughts. Then just as quickly, he'd turn back to his desk, determined to wrap up school before fatherhood consumed him.

But me? Parenthood had already preoccupied every ounce of my being. I hadn't known I could fall so in love with someone, especially a baby I'd never even met.

This inexplicable joy can thrust any of us into an amphitheater of to-do lists, grandiose milestones, tests, expectations, and external comparisons. Our glee blurs into this contagious battle of the bands where anyone—family, coworkers, a random person on the sidewalk—wants to drop in on the show and bang a drum or toot a horn. It feels so exciting! It also gets a bit nerve-wracking and noisy.

Sometimes we need to lower the volume just enough to hear the heartbeats thumping inside us. This mother-child duet is the song we're meant to hear. It's the rhythm that makes motherhood sacred.

I knew I didn't want to miss that sweet melody because I let myself become too busy being anywhere but in the moment with my unborn baby. So I bent down and rummaged through a drawer near Martin's feet, not knowing that I was about to begin something that would change my life profoundly.

"What are you looking for?" he asked, without glancing over.

"A new journal. I'm going upstairs to write our baby a love letter."

A grin filled his face as he set down his pencil and looked me in the eye. "Tell our little one I say hi."

I've always enjoyed journaling because it grants me access to the story vibrating in my heart. And I relish watching how it does that for others. Titles we give ourselves such as "I'm pregnant" acquire more depth through writing, as we slow down to reflect on the lyrics and contemplate our experiences and emotions rather than merely noting data or hearing how others tell our overture for us. Even the briefest entries about what we hope and how we feel can unlock an inner opus as powerful as Beethoven's Fifth Symphony. They help us unearth our truest personal definitions of love, beauty, joy, and anticipation—emotions that sometimes get smothered by the chaos of fear, uncertainty, and daily distractions.

Innumerable studies reveal that pregnancy journaling helps moms-to-be develop stronger attachments to our babies, ease stress, and feel more confident. When I paused to write to my baby, I rested more, like my doctor wanted. But the process developed into so much more.

My journal became a keepsake box capturing the tiniest details: the smell of freshly cut grass on the way to our first ultrasound, my obsession with olives, or the day Martin turned in his last homework assignment. It housed records of both loss and celebration in our lives, along with dozens of reminders of how much I loved my growing baby. All wrapped together, that series of letters became the most beautiful story I'd ever known. In fact, if we ever face the misfortune of losing our home to fire, I will risk flames and smoke to run in and extract that journal, because through it, I truly understood that while my baby would eventually depart my body, he would never leave my heart.

Fast forward to earlier this year when my doctor confirmed I was expecting our second child. Martin and I laughed. We cried. And we both knew I had to compose another pregnancy journal. This time, the series of love letters wouldn't just be for our baby—I needed to create a music box for you to hold the cherished song you feel for your unborn baby (and yourself) in this brief, beautiful time.

You'll find varying types of prompts throughout this journal. Some will make you rub your belly and smile, while others address topics that might feel difficult but will bring you closer to your baby. Keep these four guideposts in mind as you write. I think they'll help you feel more confident as you lean into your rich and valuable story.

1. Celebrate the depths of your feelings.

Delve into all the nooks and crannies of your joy, and fill this journal with as many hearts and "I love yous" as you fancy. When you find moments that require you to face fear, claim your strength, or accept things you can't control, give yourself permission to write your way through what you're really feeling. I know how scary it is to admit vulnerability and feelings of failure or to stay true to ideas that are uniquely yours. But I've learned that writing them down can give you the space to reflect on them calmly. Through all the challenges of life, remember that you're performing a superhero act of growing an all-new person. And through this journal you'll record the beauty of your story.

2. Let go of perfection.

One way to take possession of your story is to write like you talk. Journaling shouldn't be about designing flawless entries—it's about unearthing your truth, and sometimes that means getting a little messy.

I cross out words in my journal all the time. There are pen smudges and squished crumbs of I-don't-know-what on my pages. I've got awkward grammar and misspelled words that would disqualify me from a fourth-grade spelling bee. But I keep going. If you try to edit as you go or outline ideas before even beginning to journal, you unwittingly take away most of the raw truth and best discoveries that come from letting your pen and heart wander across the page.

You just have to start.

Flip your journal open to any page. Set a timer and write until it dings. Or pretend you're in the middle of an intimate conversation. You'll find that many of the prompts in this journal begin with sentiments such as "Dear Baby" or "Hello Little One" to help you ease into comfortable and natural storycatching.

3. Play.

Think of this journal as a pocket to your heart that holds your birdsong. Plenty of teenage girls compose notebook pages of heart doodles, bubble letters, and practice signatures in every color and glitter capacity imaginable. While it might feel tedious to dot every *i* with a heart, those adolescent gestures capture the exact romantic, hopeful feeling we have about life when we're pregnant. The process of doodling, decorating, and gathering keepsakes for your journal gives you an opportunity to reflect on your baby. So jot *xoxo* all you want! Practice writing your baby's name across the pages. Experiment with pens. Underline words or color them in. Above all, tuck in memorabilia: belly photos, ultrasound images, clothing tags, receipts, quotations, sentimental notes, screenshots, and anything else that encapsulates moments of your narrative.

4. Go beyond these pages.

Your storycatching only begins with the pages of this journal. Come join me for exclusive *Awaiting You* resources, which include unexpected ways to document milestones, motivational journaling tricks you'll love, the TEDx Talk I gave (while eight months pregnant!), and examples from my own journals online at:

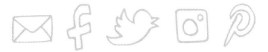

KATIECLEMONS.COM/A/VRC3

I'd love to hear how your journal is coming together. Please drop me a note at **howdy@katieclemons.com** (I answer all my mail) or join me on social media **@katierclemons**, **#katieclemonsjournals**, and **#awaitingyoujournal**.

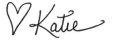

The narratives you record in this journal capture your experiences and create a keepsake for the future. Imagine opening this music box and reading these love letters in ten or twenty years, or passing it on to your grown child. Wrapped all together, the stories you write are the beginning of one of the most beautiful love songs on earth.

You're a great mom already. Sing your heart out, and... Let's celebrate your story!

♡ Katie

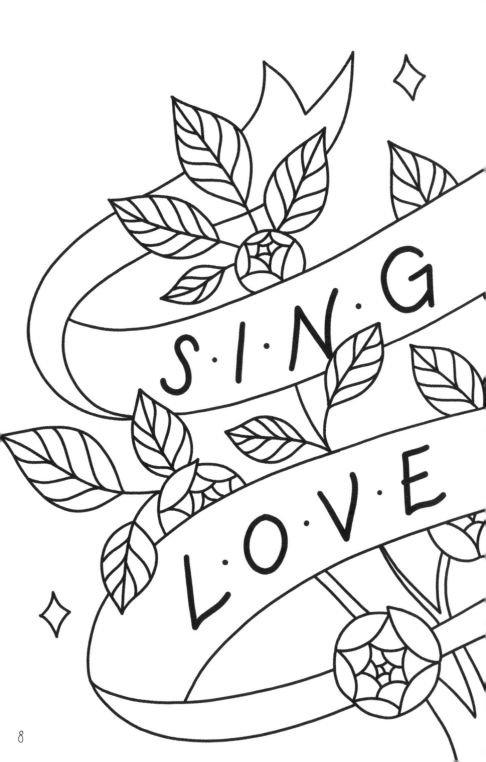

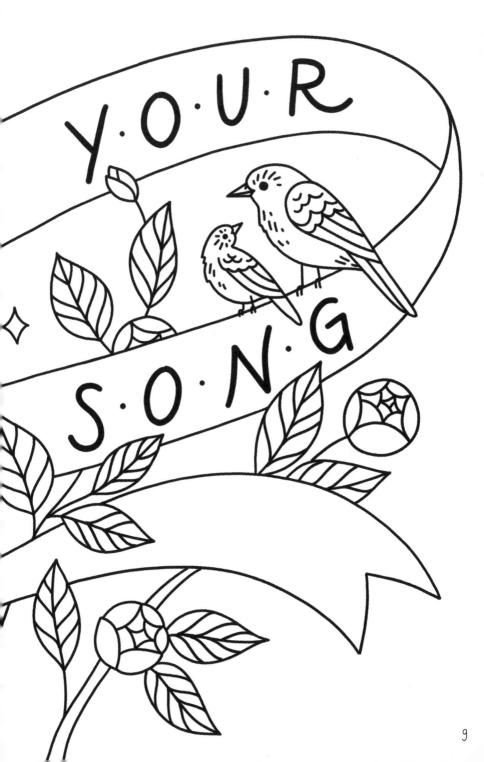

You & Me

An early pregnancy picture

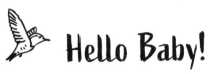

Hello Baby!

This journal chronicles moments of my pregnancy with you. The bigger you grow, the more my heart expands. I'm grateful for the gift of being your mom, and I cannot wait to hold you in my arms.

My name

My age and location

Today's date

Weeks along and due date

In my heart, I'm feeling

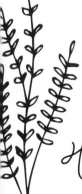

Here's how **OUR STORY BEGINS...**

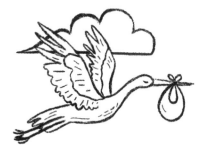

My Little One

The day I knew I was pregnant with you

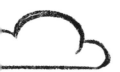

DATE _____ WEEKS ALONG _____

Sweet Baby,

I'm so happy to welcome you and love you because

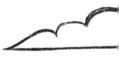

Around Here

Current national or global event worth noting

_____

_____

_____

My thoughts

_____

_____

_____

Current local event here in _____ worth noting

_____

_____

_____

My thoughts

_____

_____

_____

_____

You & Me

What I hope changes in my life after you're born

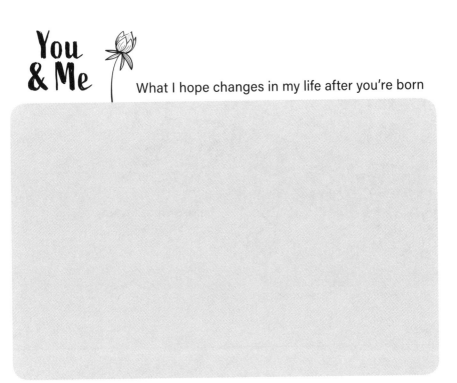

What I hope remains the same

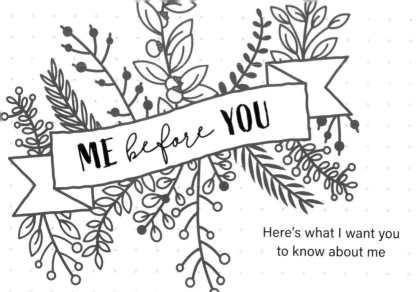

ME before YOU

Here's what I want you
to know about me

Today I am
feeling thankful for

♥

♥

♥

♥

♥

♥

♥

♥

♥

♥

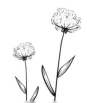

DATE _____ WEEKS ALONG _____

Sweet Baby, I got to hear your heartbeat.

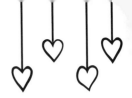

Checking In

Here are some notes from a recent prenatal care checkup
along with a few of my thoughts

Hello Baby!

Today I want to tell you about

Hello Baby!

Let me tell you about our home and everyone who lives here

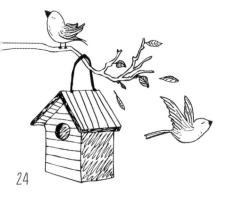

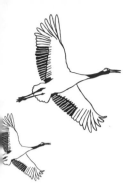

We're eager to *welcome* you home

Adhere a photo or doodle and write some details about your home and family.

Dear Baby,

I want to tell you about your daddy

_____

_____

_____

_____

_____

_____

_____

_____

_____

_____

These are traits I admire in him

1. _____

2. _____

3. _____

4. _____

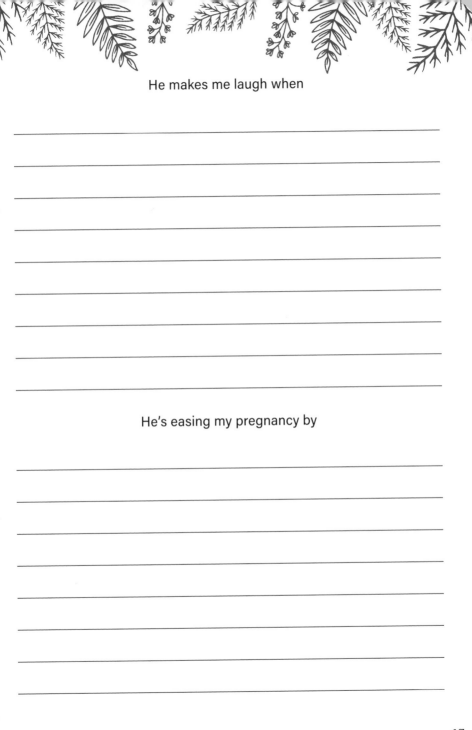

He makes me laugh when

_____

_____

_____

_____

_____

_____

_____

_____

He's easing my pregnancy by

_____

_____

_____

_____

_____

_____

_____

_____

Your Daddy & Me *before you*

We met when

At the time, he was spending a lot of time on

I was spending a lot of time on

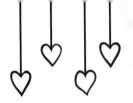

Our first date was
- - - - - - - - - - - - - - - - - -

I still remember how he
- -

I know he already loves you because
- -

I predict that when you're a baby, he'll
- -

I'll bet that when you're older, he'll really want to
- -

Come and let us love you

Ask the dad-to-be to write. Interview him.
Adhere screenshots of his texts. Or record thoughts he's shared.

Dear Baby,

This is how I told loved ones that we're awaiting your arrival

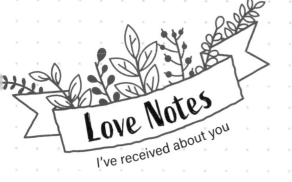

Love Notes

I've received about you

Add keepsakes here. Jot down what people have said or done. Adhere a card, drawing, or photo. Print off an email, text, or social media conversation. Or pass this page and a pen to the ones you love.

DATE _____ WEEKS ALONG _____

This Is Now

My morning routine

My end-of-the-day routine

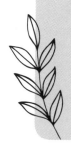

DATE _____ WEEKS ALONG _____

Hello Little One

These are my hopes for you as you grow in the world

Hello Baby!

Today I want to tell you about

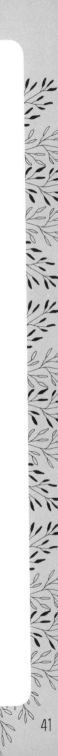

Skills and Talents
I hope you explore (and why)

DATE _____ WEEKS ALONG _____

Around Here

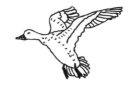

You're currently the size of

You feel more like the size of

Sleep is

You and I consume incredible amounts of

I'm looking forward to

Dear Baby,

Becoming your mom makes me feel

Add mantras,
lyrics, or words of
wisdom. Adhere
memorabilia.
Doodle. Or write
and reflect.

People I can't wait
for you to meet

Hello Baby!

This is the story of a typical dinner
scene at our home right now

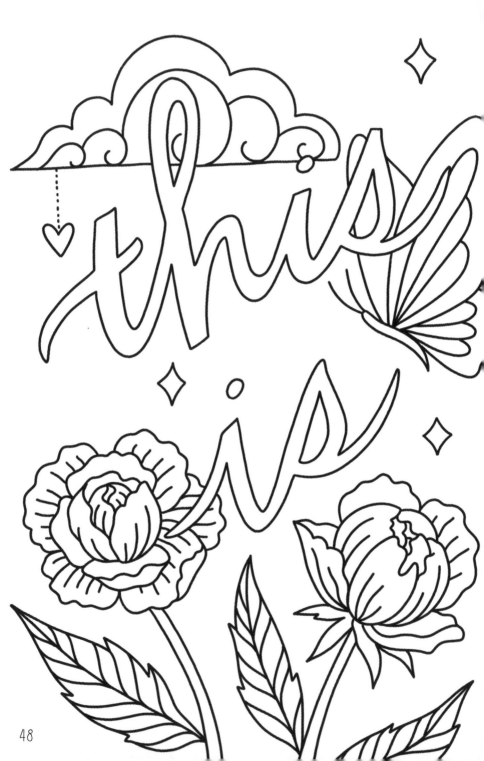

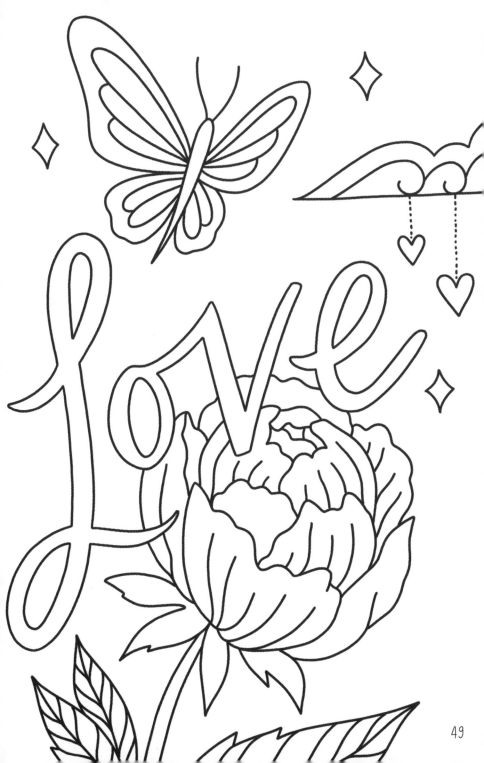

My Little Darling,

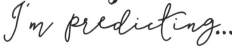

I'm predicting...

How much of my favorite pregnancy food
(_____)
I'll eat before you're born

The number of days early/late you'll arrive

Boy or girl

The number of kisses I'll give you the day you're born

How many family members you'll meet the day you're born

How many diapers we'll go through in your first week

_____

_____

_____

_____

_____

_____

_____

_____

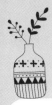

Hello Little One

A hundred things run through my mind. They're all about you.

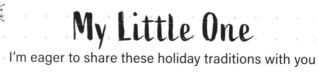

My Little One

I'm eager to share these holiday traditions with you

And I look forward to establishing
some traditions of our own

Sweet Baby,

Waiting for you is hard!

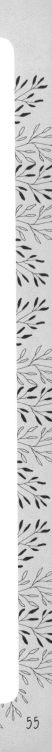

My Childhood Favorites

Books, shows, games, and toys I'm eager to share with you

♥ _____

♥ _____

♥ _____

♥ _____

♥ _____

♥ _____

♥ _____

♥ _____

♥ _____

♥ _____

♥ _____

♥ _____

DATE _____ WEEKS ALONG _____

This Is Now

My typical weekday looks like

My usual weekend looks like

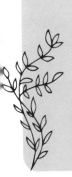

Sweet Baby,

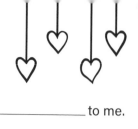

You are _____ to me.

_____

_____

_____

_____

_____

_____

_____

_____

_____

_____

_____

_____

_____

_____

_____

_____

_____

_____

_____

_____

_____

_____

_____

  DATE _____ WEEKS ALONG _____

Currently on My

· NIGHTSTAND ·

· PLAYLIST ·

· FEET ·

· WISH LIST ·

· CALENDAR ·

· BED ·

DATE _____ WEEKS ALONG _____

How I feel in my heart

courageous

grateful

hopeful

glowing

rushed

inspired

beautiful

gentle

nourished

loving

tender

frazzled

strong

loved

connected

joyful

content

forgetful

delighted

fearful

awkward

patient

fulfilled

curious

flexible

brave

upended

rested

capable

overwhelmed

nervous

Mark appropriate words.

huge

alive

hungry

Reflections
on the words I chose

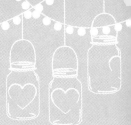

Hello Little One

Meeting you at an ultrasound felt

DATE _____ WEEKS ALONG _____

Your heart will never be alone

Add an
ultrasound
picture or other
keepsake.

Checking In

Here are some notes from a recent prenatal care checkup
along with a few of my thoughts

Small ways our home is changing for your arrival

My Little One

I bought something special for you

Sweet Baby,

I imagine who you'll become

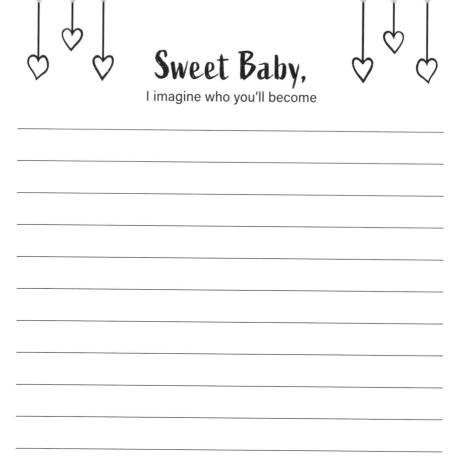

_____

_____

_____

_____

_____

_____

_____

I look forward to sharing these moments with you

♥ _____

♥ _____

♥ _____

♥ _____

These are traits that I hope describe the type of person you'll become

♥ _____

♥ _____

♥ _____

♥ _____

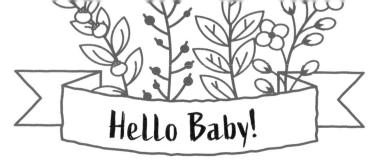

Hello Baby!

Today I want to tell you about

_____

_____

_____

_____

_____

_____

_____

_____

_____

_____

_____

_____

_____

_____

_____

_____

_____

My darling Baby,

I adore these details about you right now

I love calling you this nickname

DATE _____ WEEKS ALONG _____

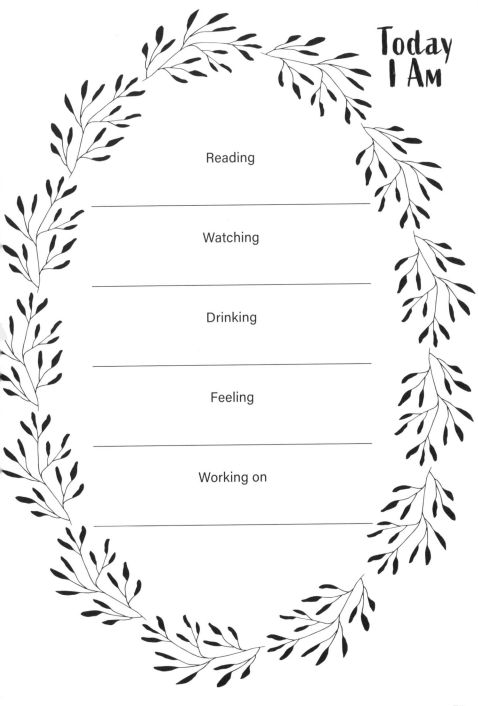

Today I Am

Reading

_____

Watching

_____

Drinking

_____

Feeling

_____

Working on

_____

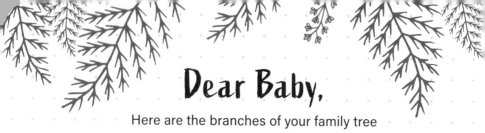

Dear Baby,

Here are the branches of your family tree

Sweet Baby,

I'm grateful _____ will be in your life because

I wish _____ could be here to watch you grow because

My little Darling,

I want to tell you about your grandparents

This Is Now

Pregnancy is transforming me into a stronger woman

It's also making me feel more vulnerable

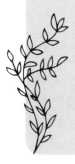

DATE _____ WEEKS ALONG _____

Hello Little One

I cherish quiet moments when it's just you and me

I always want *to remember*

Today

This week or month

This year

This imperfectly beautiful life

DATE _____ WEEKS ALONG _____

ME before YOU

Pre-motherhood accomplishments I'm proud of

1. _____

_____

_____

2. _____

_____

_____

3. _____

_____

_____

4. _____

_____

_____

Today I Am

Hoping I can emulate some choices my parents made for me when I was growing up

DATE _____ WEEKS ALONG _____

Dear Baby,

This is a story about someone who already loves you so much

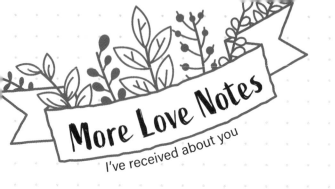

More Love Notes

I've received about you

True Love

Adhere a photo or ultrasound image.
Draw, write, or adhere a poem, letter, or keepsake.

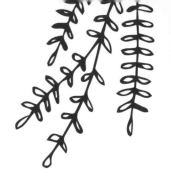

Hello Baby!

I know my heart will always adore you because

Checking In

Here are some notes from a recent prenatal care checkup
along with a few of my thoughts

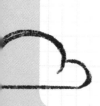

DATE _____ WEEKS ALONG _____

Right Now

Several ways you make me inexplicably happy are

♥ _____

♥ _____

♥ _____

♥ _____

I know I'm doing a GREAT JOB because

♥ _____

♥ _____

♥ _____

♥ _____

When I see another pregnant mom or a new baby

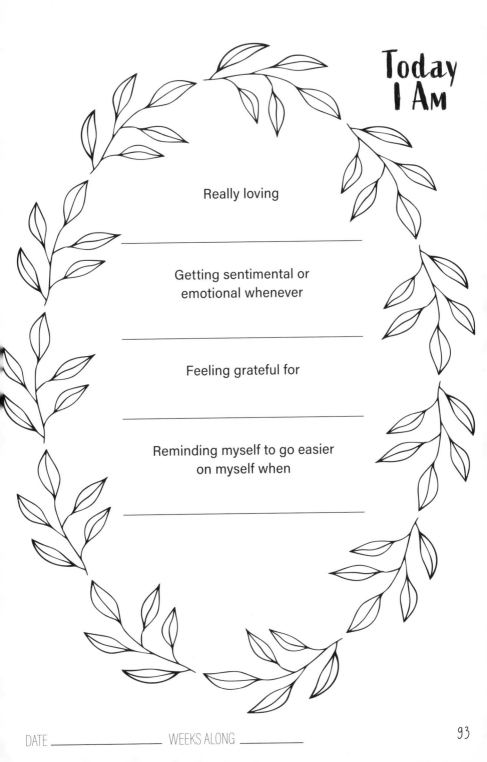

Today
I Am

Really loving

_____

Getting sentimental or
emotional whenever

_____

Feeling grateful for

_____

Reminding myself to go easier
on myself when

_____

These toys are already waiting for you to come play

DATE _____ WEEKS ALONG _____

Hello Little One

Without you, today would be an ordinary day.
You bring me such joy!

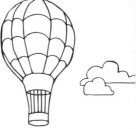

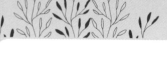

Hello Baby!

Today I want to tell you about

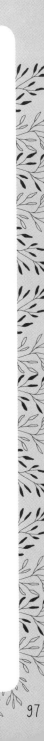

My Little Darling,

I hope you can keep this family recipe alive

Here's the story behind it

_____

_____

_____

_____

_____

_____

_____

_____

_____

_____

_____

_____

_____

_____

_____

_____

_____

_____

_____

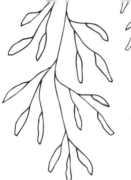

Sweet Baby,

I want you to know about trying and failing,
especially when you think you'll never achieve a dream,
because I've been there. I'll be back many times,
and I have learned that...

DATE _____ WEEKS ALONG _____

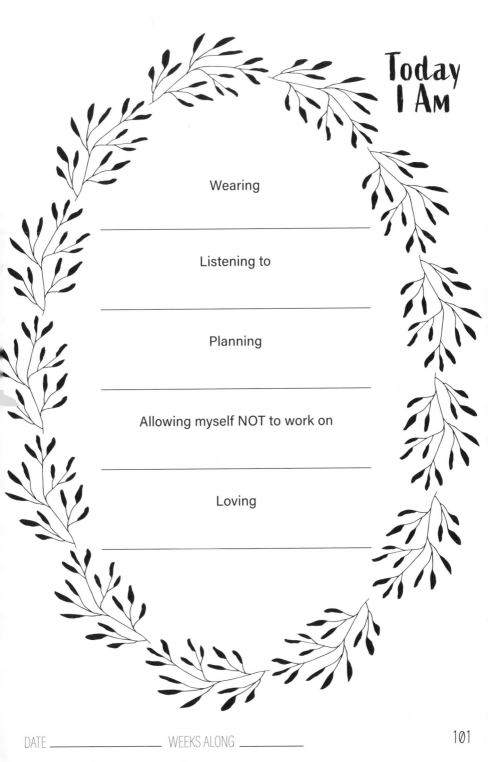

Today I Am

Wearing

_____

Listening to

_____

Planning

_____

Allowing myself NOT to work on

_____

Loving

_____

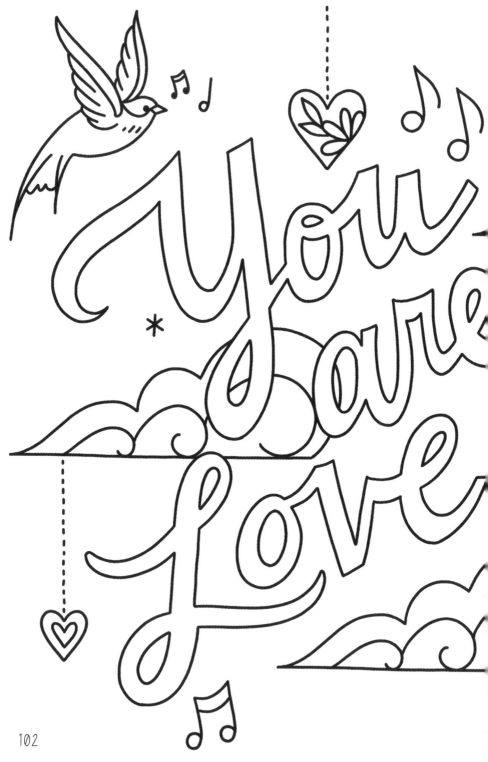

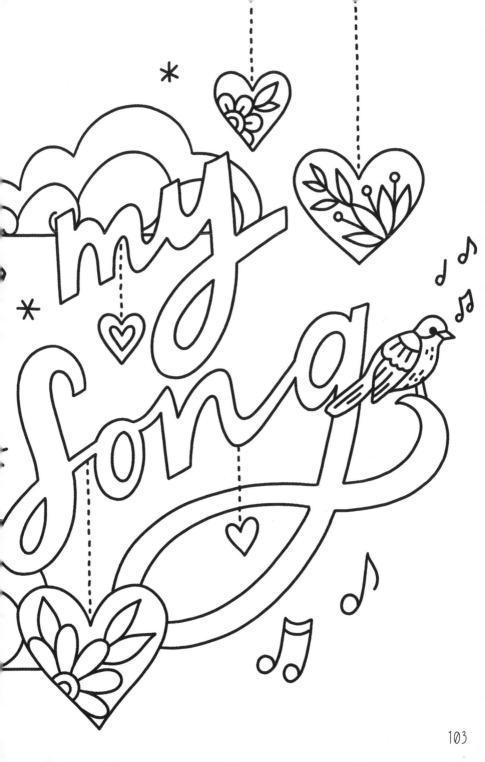

These cute clothes await your arrival

Dear Baby,

When I woke up this morning

Hello Baby!

Thinking of a name for you

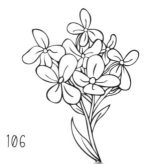

DATE _____ WEEKS ALONG _____

These books are waiting for you to read and treasure them

True Love

Adhere a photo or ultrasound image.
Draw, write, or adhere a poem, letter, or keepsake.

My Little Darling,

You and I are so lucky

Gifts and heirlooms
you are receiving

Around Here

On a scale of 1–5, I'm feeling

JOYFUL ♡ ♡ ♡ ♡ ♡

COMFORTABLE ♡ ♡ ♡ ♡ ♡

RESTED ♡ ♡ ♡ ♡ ♡

NERVOUS ♡ ♡ ♡ ♡ ♡

PATIENT ♡ ♡ ♡ ♡ ♡

HUNGRY ♡ ♡ ♡ ♡ ♡

CALM ♡ ♡ ♡ ♡ ♡

Reflections on my ratings

_____

_____

_____

_____

_____

_____

_____

_____

_____

_____

_____

_____

_____

_____

_____

_____

_____

_____

_____

_____

Dear Baby,

You are _____ .

DATE _____ WEEKS ALONG _____

My Typical Weekday

6:00 _____

7:00 _____

8:00 _____

9:00 _____

10:00 _____

11:00 _____

NOON _____

1:00 _____

2:00 _____

3:00 _____

4:00 _____

5:00 _____

6:00 _____

7:00 _____

8:00 _____

9:00 _____

10:00 _____

Discovering
Boy or Girl!

Checking In

Here are some notes from a recent prenatal care checkup
along with a few of my thoughts

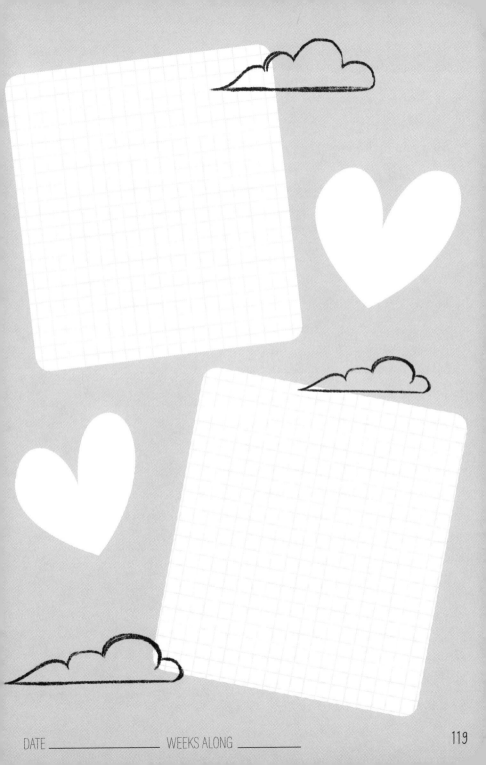

We're preparing
for your arrival

Bed and bedroom

_____

_____

_____

Car seat

_____

_____

_____

Feeding supplies

_____

_____

_____

Diapers

_____

_____

_____

Toys and books

_____

_____

_____

Clothes

_____

_____

_____

Stroller or carrier

_____

_____

_____

Bathing gear

_____

_____

_____

And of course

_____

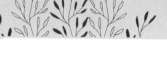

Hello Baby!

I want to tell you a happy story from my childhood

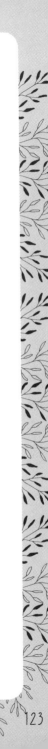

I hold you.

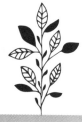

You hold my heart.

DATE _____ WEEKS ALONG _____

My Little One

With a quick rib kick or stretch, you remind me I am not alone

My Little One

I imagine our family ten years from now

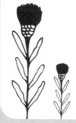

Sweet Baby,

If I could offer you one piece of advice for when
you're _____ years old like I am now

Hello Little One

I never want to forget a few details about my time pregnant with you

DATE _____ WEEKS ALONG _____

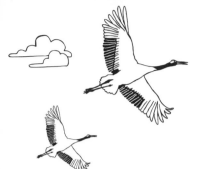

Around Here

Planning for your birth

Dear Baby,

You're coming soon!

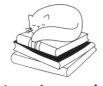

Welcome to the family

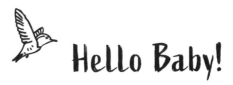

Hello Baby!

Your name

Date and time of birth

Location and weather

Height and weight

In my heart, I'm feeling

WE'VE BEEN *awaiting you*

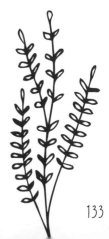

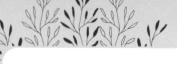

Dear Baby,

This is the story of your arrival

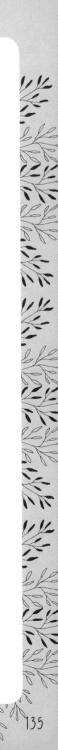

Around Here

Current national or global event worth noting

_____

_____

_____

My thoughts

_____

_____

_____

Current local event here in _____ worth noting

_____

_____

_____

My thoughts

_____

_____

_____

_____

DATE _____ DAYS OLD _____

Sweet Baby,

I will cherish these newborn moments forever

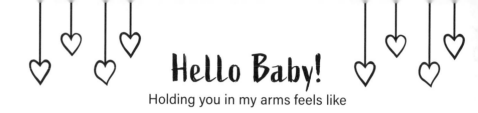

Hello Baby!

Holding you in my arms feels like

DATE _____ DAYS OLD _____

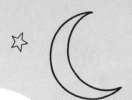

You & Me
Our sleepy faces

· MOM · **· BABY ·**

Our hungry faces

· MOM · **· BABY ·**

Our _____ faces

· MOM · **· BABY ·**

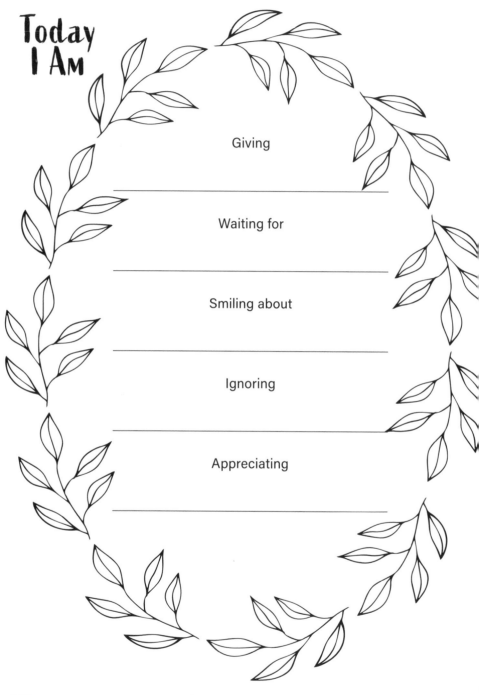

Today I Am

Giving

_____

Waiting for

_____

Smiling about

_____

Ignoring

_____

Appreciating

_____

DATE _____ DAYS OLD _____

My Typical Weekday

6:00 _____

7:00 _____

8:00 _____

9:00 _____

10:00 _____

11:00 _____

NOON _____

1:00 _____

2:00 _____

3:00 _____

4:00 _____

5:00 _____

6:00 _____

7:00 _____

8:00 _____

9:00 _____

10:00 _____

DATE _____ DAYS OLD _____

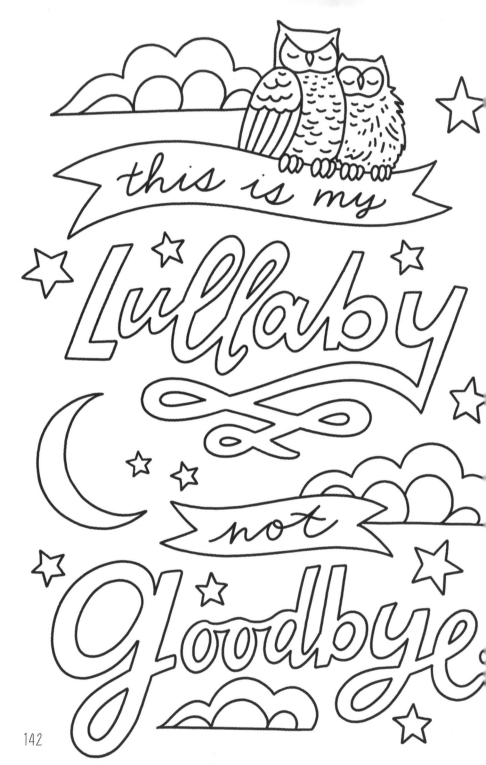

this is my

Lullaby

not

Goodbye.

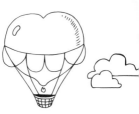

Hello Baby!

I have a few last thoughts I want to share
before I finish this journal—my love letter to you

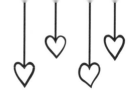

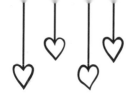

Let's Celebrate Your Story!

I believe that your story is one of the most meaningful gifts you can give yourself and the people you love. Thank you for entrusting me and this journal with your adventures. If you loved writing in these pages, let's celebrate more of your story with my other books. They're just as empowering and, well, awesome!

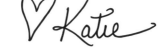

♥ **Love, Mom and Me:** A Mother & Daughter Keepsake Journal

♥ **Between Mom and Me:** A Mother & Son Keepsake Journal

♥ **Between Dad and Me:** A Father & Son Keepsake Journal

♥ **Love, Dad and Me:** A Father & Daughter Keepsake Journal

DISCOVER EVEN MORE KATIE CLEMONS JOURNALS AT KATIECLEMONS.COM!